MIRACLE DIET

TRACK YOUR DIET SUCCESS
WITH FOOD PYRAMID, CALORIE GUIDE
AND BMI CHART

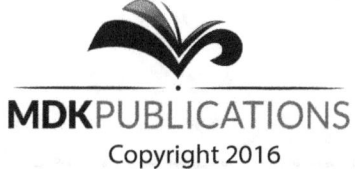

MDKPUBLICATIONS
Copyright 2016

BODY MASS INDEX

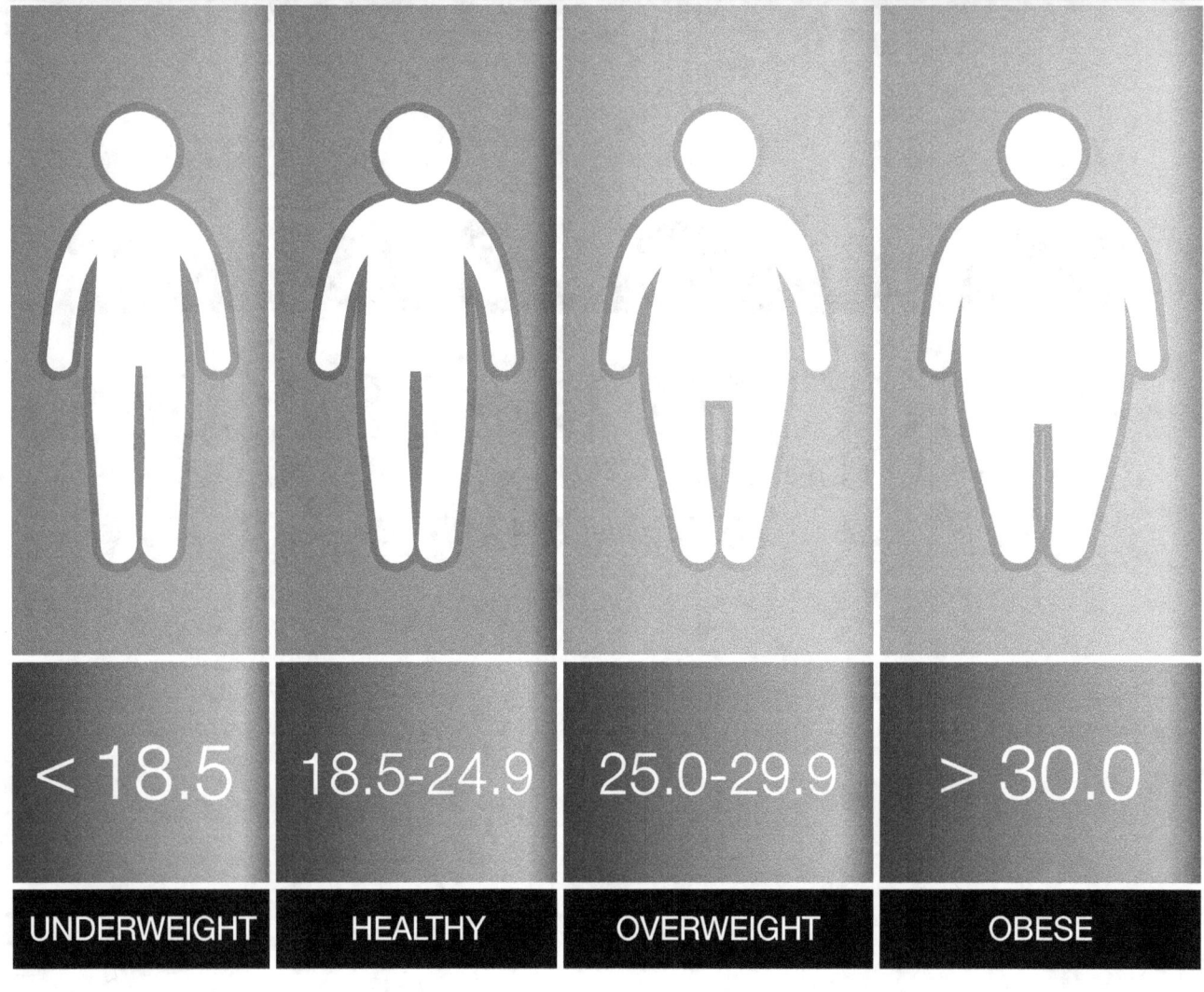

< 18.5	18.5-24.9	25.0-29.9	> 30.0
UNDERWEIGHT	HEALTHY	OVERWEIGHT	OBESE

NOTES:

_____

_____

_____

_____

_____

CALORIE IN FRUIT

∿ INFOGRAPHICS ∿

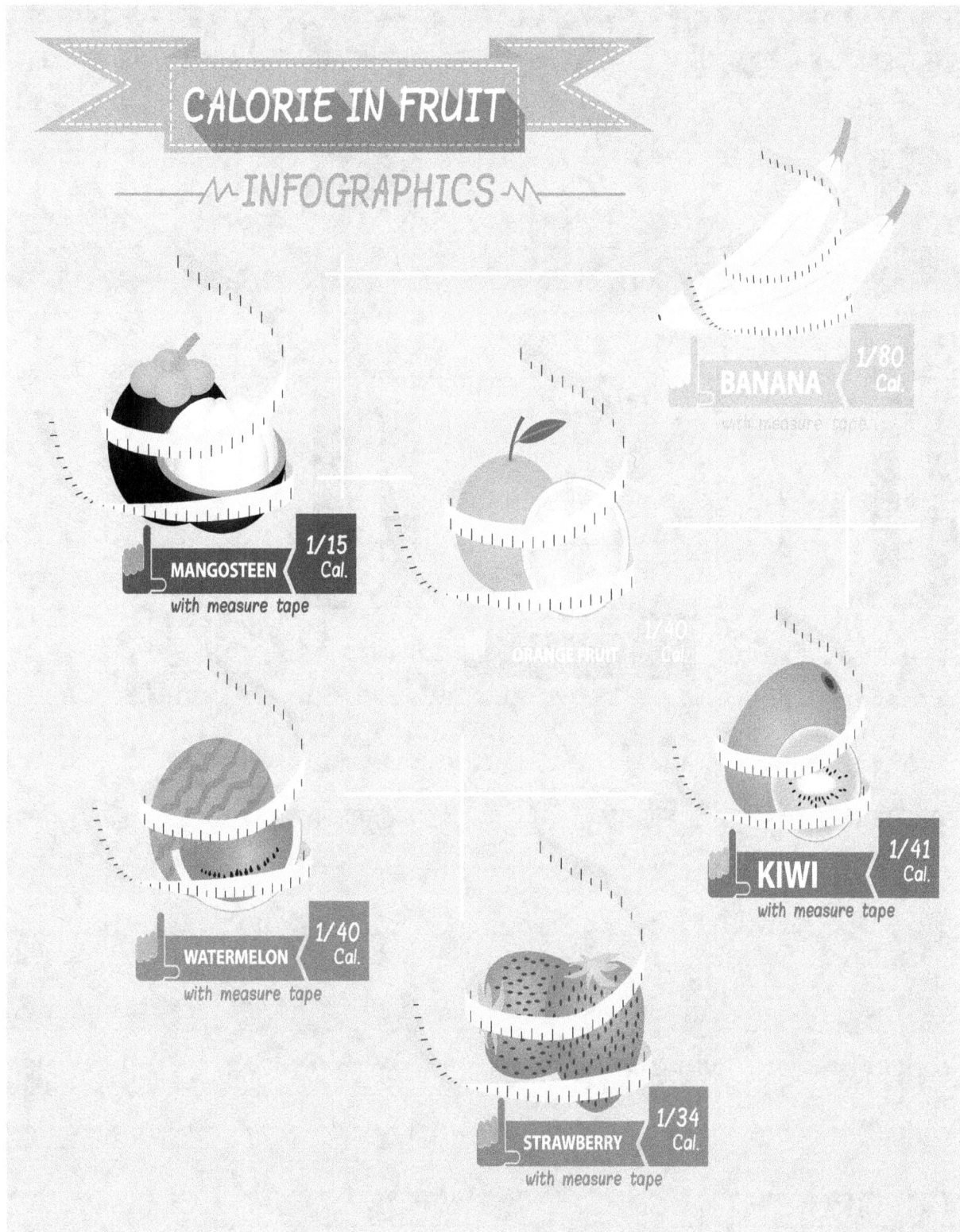

BANANA 1/80 Cal.
with measure tape

MANGOSTEEN 1/15 Cal.
with measure tape

ORANGE FRUIT 1/40 Cal.

KIWI 1/41 Cal.
with measure tape

WATERMELON 1/40 Cal.
with measure tape

STRAWBERRY 1/34 Cal.
with measure tape

TIPS:

_____

_____

_____

_____

YOU ARE WHAT YOU EAT

INFOGRAPHIC

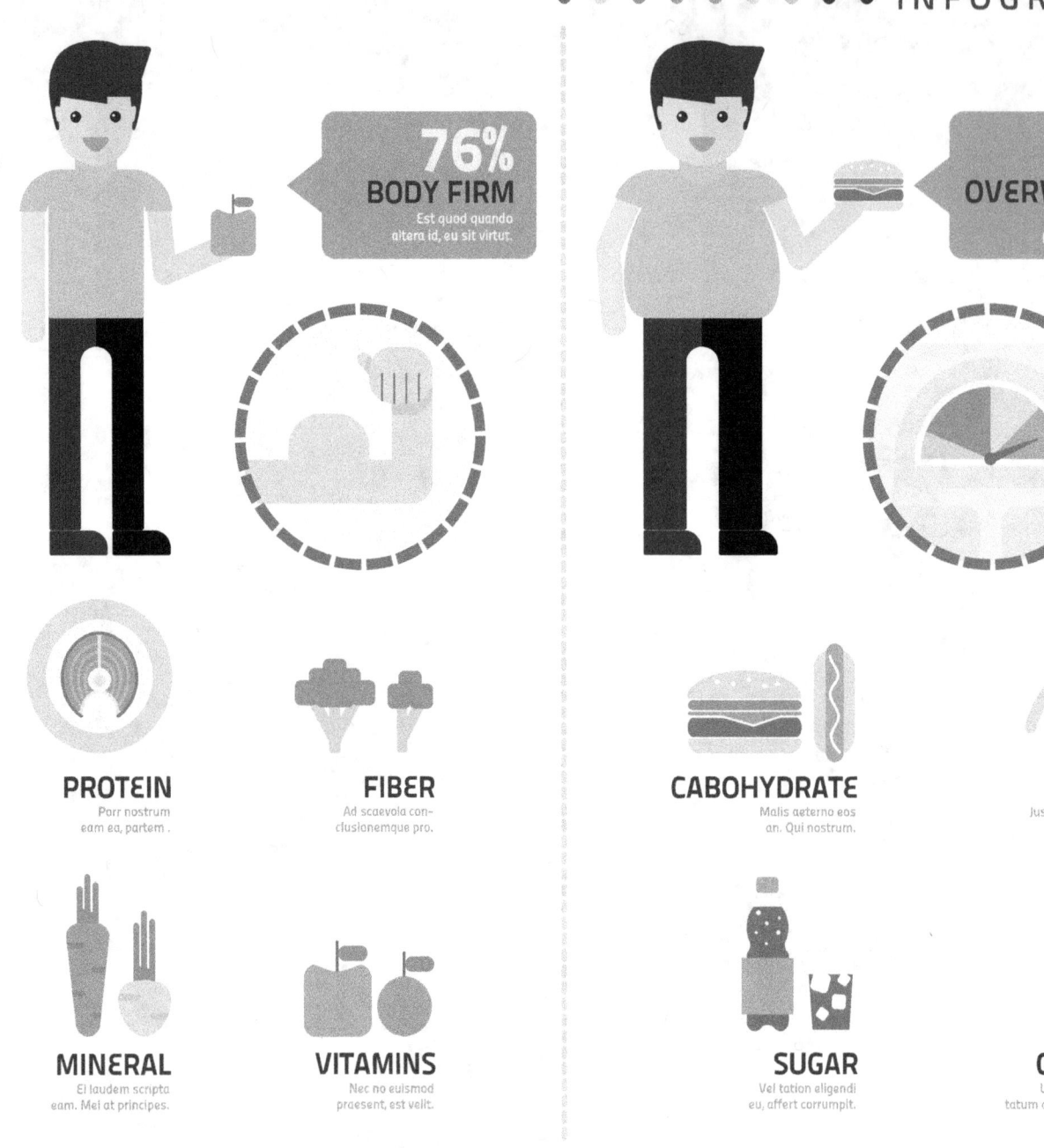

76%
BODY FIRM
Est quod quando
altera id, eu sit virtut.

89%
OVERWEIGHT
Te sint volumus
per, erant nullam.

PROTEIN
Parr nostrum
eam ea, partem .

FIBER
Ad scaevola con-
clusionemque pro.

CABOHYDRATE
Malis aeterno eos
an. Qui nostrum.

FAT
Justo veniam de-
tracto vim no.

MINERAL
El laudem scripta
eam. Mel at principes.

VITAMINS
Nec no euismod
praesent, est velit.

SUGAR
Vel tation eligendi
eu, affert corrumpit.

CREAM
Usu ignota lup-
tatum at, el eum nibh.

DON'T FORGET TO

_____

_____

_____

_____

_____

Personal Goals

Start Date: _____   **End Date:** _____

My Goal:

_____

_____

_____

_____

_____

My Plan:

_____

_____

_____

_____

_____

Daily Food Target

Calories	Fat
Carbs	Fiber
Protein	Others
TOTAL	

Physical Activity Target

Daily Activity	Qty/Time
_____	_____
_____	_____
_____	_____
_____	_____

and/or

Weekly Activity	Qty/Time
_____	_____
_____	_____
_____	_____
_____	_____

My Statistics

Goal	Record one or more	Before	After	Net +/-

DAY #:_____

Meal 1	Portion Sizes	Fat	Calories	Carbs	Protein
TOTALS					
Satisfied after eating?					

Meal 2	Portion Sizes	Fat	Calories	Carbs	Protein
TOTALS					
Satisfied after eating?					

Notes

Meal 3	Portion Sizes	Fat	Calories	Carbs	Protein
TOTALS					
Satisfied after eating?					

Meal 4	Portion Sizes	Fat	Calories	Carbs	Protein
TOTALS					
Satisfied after eating?					

Meal 5	Portion Sizes	Fat	Calories	Carbs	Protein
TOTALS					
Satisfied after eating?					

DAY #:＿＿＿＿＿＿＿＿＿

Meal 1	Portion Sizes	Fat	Calories	Carbs	Protein
TOTALS					
Satisfied after eating?					

Meal 2	Portion Sizes	Fat	Calories	Carbs	Protein
TOTALS					
Satisfied after eating?					

Notes

Meal 3	Portion Sizes	Fat	Calories	Carbs	Protein
TOTALS					

Satisfied after eating?	

Meal 4	Portion Sizes	Fat	Calories	Carbs	Protein
TOTALS					

Satisfied after eating?	

Meal 5	Portion Sizes	Fat	Calories	Carbs	Protein
TOTALS					

Satisfied after eating?	

DAY #: _____

Meal 1	Portion Sizes	Fat	Calories	Carbs	Protein
TOTALS					

Satisfied after eating?

Meal 2	Portion Sizes	Fat	Calories	Carbs	Protein
TOTALS					

Satisfied after eating?

Notes

Meal 3	Portion Sizes	Fat	Calories	Carbs	Protein
TOTALS					

Satisfied after eating?	

Meal 4	Portion Sizes	Fat	Calories	Carbs	Protein
TOTALS					

Satisfied after eating?	

Meal 5	Portion Sizes	Fat	Calories	Carbs	Protein
TOTALS					

Satisfied after eating?	

DAY #:_____

Meal 1	Portion Sizes	Fat	Calories	Carbs	Protein
TOTALS					

Satisfied after eating? ⬚

Meal 2	Portion Sizes	Fat	Calories	Carbs	Protein
TOTALS					

Satisfied after eating? ⬚

Notes

Meal 3	Portion Sizes	Fat	Calories	Carbs	Protein
TOTALS					

Satisfied after eating?	

Meal 4	Portion Sizes	Fat	Calories	Carbs	Protein
TOTALS					

Satisfied after eating?	

Meal 5	Portion Sizes	Fat	Calories	Carbs	Protein
TOTALS					

Satisfied after eating?	

DAY #: _____

Meal 1	Portion Sizes	Fat	Calories	Carbs	Protein
TOTALS					
Satisfied after eating?					

Meal 2	Portion Sizes	Fat	Calories	Carbs	Protein
TOTALS					
Satisfied after eating?					

Notes

Meal 3	Portion Sizes	Fat	Calories	Carbs	Protein
TOTALS					
Satisfied after eating?					

Meal 4	Portion Sizes	Fat	Calories	Carbs	Protein
TOTALS					
Satisfied after eating?					

Meal 5	Portion Sizes	Fat	Calories	Carbs	Protein
TOTALS					
Satisfied after eating?					

DAY #:_____

Meal 1	Portion Sizes	Fat	Calories	Carbs	Protein
TOTALS					

Satisfied after eating?	

Meal 2	Portion Sizes	Fat	Calories	Carbs	Protein
TOTALS					

Satisfied after eating?	

Notes

Meal 3	Portion Sizes		Fat	Calories	Carbs	Protein
TOTALS						
Satisfied after eating?						

Meal 4	Portion Sizes		Fat	Calories	Carbs	Protein
TOTALS						
Satisfied after eating?						

Meal 5	Portion Sizes		Fat	Calories	Carbs	Protein
TOTALS						
Satisfied after eating?						

DAY #:_____

Meal 1	Portion Sizes	Fat	Calories	Carbs	Protein
TOTALS					

Satisfied after eating?

Meal 2	Portion Sizes	Fat	Calories	Carbs	Protein
TOTALS					

Satisfied after eating?

Notes

Meal 3	Portion Sizes	Fat	Calories	Carbs	Protein
TOTALS					

Satisfied after eating? ⬭

Meal 4	Portion Sizes	Fat	Calories	Carbs	Protein
TOTALS					

Satisfied after eating? ⬭

Meal 5	Portion Sizes	Fat	Calories	Carbs	Protein
TOTALS					

Satisfied after eating? ⬭

DAY #: _____

Meal 1	Portion Sizes	Fat	Calories	Carbs	Protein
TOTALS					

Satisfied after eating? ⬚

Meal 2	Portion Sizes	Fat	Calories	Carbs	Protein
TOTALS					

Satisfied after eating? ⬚

Notes

Meal 3	Portion Sizes	Fat	Calories	Carbs	Protein
TOTALS					

Satisfied after eating?	

Meal 4	Portion Sizes	Fat	Calories	Carbs	Protein
TOTALS					

Satisfied after eating?	

Meal 5	Portion Sizes	Fat	Calories	Carbs	Protein
TOTALS					

Satisfied after eating?	

DAY #:_____

Meal 1	Portion Sizes	Fat	Calories	Carbs	Protein
TOTALS					

Satisfied after eating? ⬭

Meal 2	Portion Sizes	Fat	Calories	Carbs	Protein
TOTALS					

Satisfied after eating? ⬭

Notes

Meal 3	Portion Sizes	Fat	Calories	Carbs	Protein
TOTALS					

Satisfied after eating?

Meal 4	Portion Sizes	Fat	Calories	Carbs	Protein
TOTALS					

Satisfied after eating?

Meal 5	Portion Sizes	Fat	Calories	Carbs	Protein
TOTALS					

Satisfied after eating?

DAY #: _____

Meal 1	Portion Sizes	Fat	Calories	Carbs	Protein
TOTALS					
Satisfied after eating?					

Meal 2	Portion Sizes	Fat	Calories	Carbs	Protein
TOTALS					
Satisfied after eating?					

Notes

Meal 3	Portion Sizes	Fat	Calories	Carbs	Protein
TOTALS					

Satisfied after eating?	

Meal 4	Portion Sizes	Fat	Calories	Carbs	Protein
TOTALS					

Satisfied after eating?	

Meal 5	Portion Sizes	Fat	Calories	Carbs	Protein
TOTALS					

Satisfied after eating?	

DAY #: _____

Meal 1	Portion Sizes	Fat	Calories	Carbs	Protein
TOTALS					

Satisfied after eating?	

Meal 2	Portion Sizes	Fat	Calories	Carbs	Protein
TOTALS					

Satisfied after eating?	

Notes

Meal 3	Portion Sizes	Fat	Calories	Carbs	Protein
TOTALS					

Satisfied after eating?	

Meal 4	Portion Sizes	Fat	Calories	Carbs	Protein
TOTALS					

Satisfied after eating?	

Meal 5	Portion Sizes	Fat	Calories	Carbs	Protein
TOTALS					

Satisfied after eating?	

DAY #:_____

Meal 1	Portion Sizes	Fat	Calories	Carbs	Protein
TOTALS					
Satisfied after eating?					

Meal 2	Portion Sizes	Fat	Calories	Carbs	Protein
TOTALS					
Satisfied after eating?					

Notes

Meal 3	Portion Sizes	Fat	Calories	Carbs	Protein
TOTALS					

Satisfied after eating?

Meal 4	Portion Sizes	Fat	Calories	Carbs	Protein
TOTALS					

Satisfied after eating?

Meal 5	Portion Sizes	Fat	Calories	Carbs	Protein
TOTALS					

Satisfied after eating?

DAY #: _____

Meal 1	Portion Sizes	Fat	Calories	Carbs	Protein
TOTALS					

Satisfied after eating? ⸤ ⸣

Meal 2	Portion Sizes	Fat	Calories	Carbs	Protein
TOTALS					

Satisfied after eating? ⸤ ⸣

Notes

Meal 3	Portion Sizes	Fat	Calories	Carbs	Protein
TOTALS					

Satisfied after eating?		

Meal 4	Portion Sizes	Fat	Calories	Carbs	Protein
TOTALS					

Satisfied after eating?		

Meal 5	Portion Sizes	Fat	Calories	Carbs	Protein
TOTALS					

Satisfied after eating?		

DAY #:_____

Meal 1	Portion Sizes	Fat	Calories	Carbs	Protein
TOTALS					
Satisfied after eating?					

Meal 2	Portion Sizes	Fat	Calories	Carbs	Protein
TOTALS					
Satisfied after eating?					

Notes

Meal 3	Portion Sizes	Fat	Calories	Carbs	Protein
TOTALS					

Satisfied after eating?

Meal 4	Portion Sizes	Fat	Calories	Carbs	Protein
TOTALS					

Satisfied after eating?

Meal 5	Portion Sizes	Fat	Calories	Carbs	Protein
TOTALS					

Satisfied after eating?

DAY #:_____

Meal 1	Portion Sizes	Fat	Calories	Carbs	Protein
TOTALS					
Satisfied after eating?					

Meal 2	Portion Sizes	Fat	Calories	Carbs	Protein
TOTALS					
Satisfied after eating?					

Notes

Meal 3	Portion Sizes	Fat	Calories	Carbs	Protein
TOTALS					
Satisfied after eating?					

Meal 4	Portion Sizes	Fat	Calories	Carbs	Protein
TOTALS					
Satisfied after eating?					

Meal 5	Portion Sizes	Fat	Calories	Carbs	Protein
TOTALS					
Satisfied after eating?					

DAY #: _____

Meal 1	Portion Sizes	Fat	Calories	Carbs	Protein
TOTALS					

Satisfied after eating? ⬭

Meal 2	Portion Sizes	Fat	Calories	Carbs	Protein
TOTALS					

Satisfied after eating? ⬭

Notes

Meal 3	Portion Sizes	Fat	Calories	Carbs	Protein
TOTALS					

Satisfied after eating?

Meal 4	Portion Sizes	Fat	Calories	Carbs	Protein
TOTALS					

Satisfied after eating?

Meal 5	Portion Sizes	Fat	Calories	Carbs	Protein
TOTALS					

Satisfied after eating?

DAY #: _____

Meal 1	Portion Sizes	Fat	Calories	Carbs	Protein
TOTALS					
Satisfied after eating?					

Meal 2	Portion Sizes	Fat	Calories	Carbs	Protein
TOTALS					
Satisfied after eating?					

Notes

Meal 3	Portion Sizes	Fat	Calories	Carbs	Protein
TOTALS					

Satisfied after eating?		

Meal 4	Portion Sizes	Fat	Calories	Carbs	Protein
TOTALS					

Satisfied after eating?		

Meal 5	Portion Sizes	Fat	Calories	Carbs	Protein
TOTALS					

Satisfied after eating?		

DAY #: _____

Meal 1	Portion Sizes	Fat	Calories	Carbs	Protein
TOTALS					
Satisfied after eating?					

Meal 2	Portion Sizes	Fat	Calories	Carbs	Protein
TOTALS					
Satisfied after eating?					

Notes

Meal 3	Portion Sizes		Fat	Calories	Carbs	Protein
TOTALS						

Satisfied after eating?

Meal 4	Portion Sizes		Fat	Calories	Carbs	Protein
TOTALS						

Satisfied after eating?

Meal 5	Portion Sizes		Fat	Calories	Carbs	Protein
TOTALS						

Satisfied after eating?

DAY #: _____

Meal 1	Portion Sizes	Fat	Calories	Carbs	Protein
TOTALS					
Satisfied after eating?					

Meal 2	Portion Sizes	Fat	Calories	Carbs	Protein
TOTALS					
Satisfied after eating?					

Notes

Meal 3	Portion Sizes	Fat	Calories	Carbs	Protein
TOTALS					
Satisfied after eating?					

Meal 4	Portion Sizes	Fat	Calories	Carbs	Protein
TOTALS					
Satisfied after eating?					

Meal 5	Portion Sizes	Fat	Calories	Carbs	Protein
TOTALS					
Satisfied after eating?					

DAY #:_____

Meal 1	Portion Sizes	Fat	Calories	Carbs	Protein
TOTALS					
Satisfied after eating?					

Meal 2	Portion Sizes	Fat	Calories	Carbs	Protein
TOTALS					
Satisfied after eating?					

Notes

Meal 3	Portion Sizes	Fat	Calories	Carbs	Protein
TOTALS					
Satisfied after eating?					

Meal 4	Portion Sizes	Fat	Calories	Carbs	Protein
TOTALS					
Satisfied after eating?					

Meal 5	Portion Sizes	Fat	Calories	Carbs	Protein
TOTALS					
Satisfied after eating?					

DAY #:_____

Meal 1	Portion Sizes	Fat	Calories	Carbs	Protein
TOTALS					
Satisfied after eating?					

Meal 2	Portion Sizes	Fat	Calories	Carbs	Protein
TOTALS					
Satisfied after eating?					

Notes

Meal 3	Portion Sizes	Fat	Calories	Carbs	Protein
TOTALS					

Satisfied after eating?	

Meal 4	Portion Sizes	Fat	Calories	Carbs	Protein
TOTALS					

Satisfied after eating?	

Meal 5	Portion Sizes	Fat	Calories	Carbs	Protein
TOTALS					

Satisfied after eating?	

DAY #: _____

Meal 1	Portion Sizes	Fat	Calories	Carbs	Protein
TOTALS					
Satisfied after eating?					

Meal 2	Portion Sizes	Fat	Calories	Carbs	Protein
TOTALS					
Satisfied after eating?					

Notes

Meal 3	Portion Sizes	Fat	Calories	Carbs	Protein
TOTALS					
Satisfied after eating?					

Meal 4	Portion Sizes	Fat	Calories	Carbs	Protein
TOTALS					
Satisfied after eating?					

Meal 5	Portion Sizes	Fat	Calories	Carbs	Protein
TOTALS					
Satisfied after eating?					

DAY #:_____

Meal 1	Portion Sizes	Fat	Calories	Carbs	Protein
TOTALS					
Satisfied after eating?					

Meal 2	Portion Sizes	Fat	Calories	Carbs	Protein
TOTALS					
Satisfied after eating?					

Notes

Meal 3	Portion Sizes	Fat	Calories	Carbs	Protein
TOTALS					
Satisfied after eating?					

Meal 4	Portion Sizes	Fat	Calories	Carbs	Protein
TOTALS					
Satisfied after eating?					

Meal 5	Portion Sizes	Fat	Calories	Carbs	Protein
TOTALS					
Satisfied after eating?					

DAY #: _____

Meal 1	Portion Sizes	Fat	Calories	Carbs	Protein
TOTALS					

Satisfied after eating? ( )

Meal 2	Portion Sizes	Fat	Calories	Carbs	Protein
TOTALS					

Satisfied after eating? ( )

Notes

Meal 3	Portion Sizes	Fat	Calories	Carbs	Protein
TOTALS					

Satisfied after eating?

Meal 4	Portion Sizes	Fat	Calories	Carbs	Protein
TOTALS					

Satisfied after eating?

Meal 5	Portion Sizes	Fat	Calories	Carbs	Protein
TOTALS					

Satisfied after eating?

DAY #: _____

Meal 1	Portion Sizes	Fat	Calories	Carbs	Protein
TOTALS					

Satisfied after eating? (...............)

Meal 2	Portion Sizes	Fat	Calories	Carbs	Protein
TOTALS					

Satisfied after eating? (...............)

Notes

Meal 3	Portion Sizes	Fat	Calories	Carbs	Protein
TOTALS					

Satisfied after eating?	

Meal 4	Portion Sizes	Fat	Calories	Carbs	Protein
TOTALS					

Satisfied after eating?	

Meal 5	Portion Sizes	Fat	Calories	Carbs	Protein
TOTALS					

Satisfied after eating?	

DAY #:_____

Meal 1	Portion Sizes	Fat	Calories	Carbs	Protein
TOTALS					

Satisfied after eating? ⬭

Meal 2	Portion Sizes	Fat	Calories	Carbs	Protein
TOTALS					

Satisfied after eating? ⬭

Notes

Meal 3	Portion Sizes	Fat	Calories	Carbs	Protein
TOTALS					

Satisfied after eating?	

Meal 4	Portion Sizes	Fat	Calories	Carbs	Protein
TOTALS					

Satisfied after eating?	

Meal 5	Portion Sizes	Fat	Calories	Carbs	Protein
TOTALS					

Satisfied after eating?	

DAY #: _____

Meal 1	Portion Sizes	Fat	Calories	Carbs	Protein
TOTALS					
Satisfied after eating?					

Meal 2	Portion Sizes	Fat	Calories	Carbs	Protein
TOTALS					
Satisfied after eating?					

Notes

Meal 3	Portion Sizes	Fat	Calories	Carbs	Protein
TOTALS					
Satisfied after eating?					

Meal 4	Portion Sizes	Fat	Calories	Carbs	Protein
TOTALS					
Satisfied after eating?					

Meal 5	Portion Sizes	Fat	Calories	Carbs	Protein
TOTALS					
Satisfied after eating?					

DAY #:_____

Meal 1	Portion Sizes	Fat	Calories	Carbs	Protein
TOTALS					
Satisfied after eating?					

Meal 2	Portion Sizes	Fat	Calories	Carbs	Protein
TOTALS					
Satisfied after eating?					

Notes

Meal 3	Portion Sizes	Fat	Calories	Carbs	Protein
TOTALS					

Satisfied after eating?

Meal 4	Portion Sizes	Fat	Calories	Carbs	Protein
TOTALS					

Satisfied after eating?

Meal 5	Portion Sizes	Fat	Calories	Carbs	Protein
TOTALS					

Satisfied after eating?

DAY #: _____

Meal 1	Portion Sizes	Fat	Calories	Carbs	Protein
TOTALS					
Satisfied after eating?					

Meal 2	Portion Sizes	Fat	Calories	Carbs	Protein
TOTALS					
Satisfied after eating?					

Notes

Meal 3	Portion Sizes	Fat	Calories	Carbs	Protein
TOTALS					

Satisfied after eating?	

Meal 4	Portion Sizes	Fat	Calories	Carbs	Protein
TOTALS					

Satisfied after eating?	

Meal 5	Portion Sizes	Fat	Calories	Carbs	Protein
TOTALS					

Satisfied after eating?	

DAY #:_____

Meal 1	Portion Sizes	Fat	Calories	Carbs	Protein
TOTALS					
Satisfied after eating?					

Meal 2	Portion Sizes	Fat	Calories	Carbs	Protein
TOTALS					
Satisfied after eating?					

Notes

Meal 3	Portion Sizes	Fat	Calories	Carbs	Protein
TOTALS					

Satisfied after eating?	

Meal 4	Portion Sizes	Fat	Calories	Carbs	Protein
TOTALS					

Satisfied after eating?	

Meal 5	Portion Sizes	Fat	Calories	Carbs	Protein
TOTALS					

Satisfied after eating?	

DAY #: _____

Meal 1	Portion Sizes	Fat	Calories	Carbs	Protein
TOTALS					

Satisfied after eating? (....................)

Meal 2	Portion Sizes	Fat	Calories	Carbs	Protein
TOTALS					

Satisfied after eating? (....................)

Notes

Meal 3	Portion Sizes	Fat	Calories	Carbs	Protein
TOTALS					

Satisfied after eating?		

Meal 4	Portion Sizes	Fat	Calories	Carbs	Protein
TOTALS					

Satisfied after eating?		

Meal 5	Portion Sizes	Fat	Calories	Carbs	Protein
TOTALS					

Satisfied after eating?		

DAY #:_____

Meal 1	Portion Sizes	Fat	Calories	Carbs	Protein
TOTALS					
Satisfied after eating?					

Meal 2	Portion Sizes	Fat	Calories	Carbs	Protein
TOTALS					
Satisfied after eating?					

Notes

Meal 3	Portion Sizes	Fat	Calories	Carbs	Protein
TOTALS					
Satisfied after eating?					

Meal 4	Portion Sizes	Fat	Calories	Carbs	Protein
TOTALS					
Satisfied after eating?					

Meal 5	Portion Sizes	Fat	Calories	Carbs	Protein
TOTALS					
Satisfied after eating?					

DAY #:_____

Meal 1	Portion Sizes	Fat	Calories	Carbs	Protein
TOTALS					

Satisfied after eating?

Meal 2	Portion Sizes	Fat	Calories	Carbs	Protein
TOTALS					

Satisfied after eating?

Notes

Meal 3	Portion Sizes	Fat	Calories	Carbs	Protein
TOTALS					
Satisfied after eating?					

Meal 4	Portion Sizes	Fat	Calories	Carbs	Protein
TOTALS					
Satisfied after eating?					

Meal 5	Portion Sizes	Fat	Calories	Carbs	Protein
TOTALS					
Satisfied after eating?					

DAY #:_____

Meal 1	Portion Sizes	Fat	Calories	Carbs	Protein
TOTALS					
Satisfied after eating?					

Meal 2	Portion Sizes	Fat	Calories	Carbs	Protein
TOTALS					
Satisfied after eating?					

Notes

Meal 3	Portion Sizes	Fat	Calories	Carbs	Protein
TOTALS					

Satisfied after eating?

Meal 4	Portion Sizes	Fat	Calories	Carbs	Protein
TOTALS					

Satisfied after eating?

Meal 5	Portion Sizes	Fat	Calories	Carbs	Protein
TOTALS					

Satisfied after eating?

DAY #: _____

Meal 1	Portion Sizes	Fat	Calories	Carbs	Protein
TOTALS					
Satisfied after eating?					

Meal 2	Portion Sizes	Fat	Calories	Carbs	Protein
TOTALS					
Satisfied after eating?					

Notes

Meal 3	Portion Sizes		Fat	Calories	Carbs	Protein
TOTALS						
Satisfied after eating?						

Meal 4	Portion Sizes		Fat	Calories	Carbs	Protein
TOTALS						
Satisfied after eating?						

Meal 5	Portion Sizes		Fat	Calories	Carbs	Protein
TOTALS						
Satisfied after eating?						

DAY #:_____

Meal 1	Portion Sizes	Fat	Calories	Carbs	Protein
TOTALS					
Satisfied after eating?					

Meal 2	Portion Sizes	Fat	Calories	Carbs	Protein
TOTALS					
Satisfied after eating?					

Notes

Meal 3	Portion Sizes	Fat	Calories	Carbs	Protein
TOTALS					

Satisfied after eating?	

Meal 4	Portion Sizes	Fat	Calories	Carbs	Protein
TOTALS					

Satisfied after eating?	

Meal 5	Portion Sizes	Fat	Calories	Carbs	Protein
TOTALS					

Satisfied after eating?	

DAY #:_____

Meal 1	Portion Sizes	Fat	Calories	Carbs	Protein
TOTALS					
Satisfied after eating?					

Meal 2	Portion Sizes	Fat	Calories	Carbs	Protein
TOTALS					
Satisfied after eating?					

Notes

Meal 3	Portion Sizes	Fat	Calories	Carbs	Protein
TOTALS					

Satisfied after eating? ⬭

Meal 4	Portion Sizes	Fat	Calories	Carbs	Protein
TOTALS					

Satisfied after eating? ⬭

Meal 5	Portion Sizes	Fat	Calories	Carbs	Protein
TOTALS					

Satisfied after eating? ⬭

DAY #:_____

Meal 1	Portion Sizes		Fat	Calories	Carbs	Protein
TOTALS						
Satisfied after eating?						

Meal 2	Portion Sizes		Fat	Calories	Carbs	Protein
TOTALS						
Satisfied after eating?						

Notes

Meal 3	Portion Sizes	Fat	Calories	Carbs	Protein
TOTALS					
Satisfied after eating?					

Meal 4	Portion Sizes	Fat	Calories	Carbs	Protein
TOTALS					
Satisfied after eating?					

Meal 5	Portion Sizes	Fat	Calories	Carbs	Protein
TOTALS					
Satisfied after eating?					

DAY #: _____

Meal 1	Portion Sizes	Fat	Calories	Carbs	Protein
TOTALS					
Satisfied after eating?					

Meal 2	Portion Sizes	Fat	Calories	Carbs	Protein
TOTALS					
Satisfied after eating?					

Notes

Meal 3	Portion Sizes	Fat	Calories	Carbs	Protein
TOTALS					
Satisfied after eating?					

Meal 4	Portion Sizes	Fat	Calories	Carbs	Protein
TOTALS					
Satisfied after eating?					

Meal 5	Portion Sizes	Fat	Calories	Carbs	Protein
TOTALS					
Satisfied after eating?					

DAY #:_____

Meal 1	Portion Sizes	Fat	Calories	Carbs	Protein
TOTALS					
Satisfied after eating?					

Meal 2	Portion Sizes	Fat	Calories	Carbs	Protein
TOTALS					
Satisfied after eating?					

Notes

Meal 3	Portion Sizes	Fat	Calories	Carbs	Protein
TOTALS					

Satisfied after eating?

Meal 4	Portion Sizes	Fat	Calories	Carbs	Protein
TOTALS					

Satisfied after eating?

Meal 5	Portion Sizes	Fat	Calories	Carbs	Protein
TOTALS					

Satisfied after eating?

DAY #: _____

Meal 1	Portion Sizes	Fat	Calories	Carbs	Protein
TOTALS					

Satisfied after eating?

Meal 2	Portion Sizes	Fat	Calories	Carbs	Protein
TOTALS					

Satisfied after eating?

Notes

Meal 3	Portion Sizes	Fat	Calories	Carbs	Protein
TOTALS					

Satisfied after eating?

Meal 4	Portion Sizes	Fat	Calories	Carbs	Protein
TOTALS					

Satisfied after eating?

Meal 5	Portion Sizes	Fat	Calories	Carbs	Protein
TOTALS					

Satisfied after eating?

DAY #:_____

Meal 1	Portion Sizes	Fat	Calories	Carbs	Protein
TOTALS					

Satisfied after eating?

Meal 2	Portion Sizes	Fat	Calories	Carbs	Protein
TOTALS					

Satisfied after eating?

Notes

Meal 3	Portion Sizes	Fat	Calories	Carbs	Protein
TOTALS					

Satisfied after eating?	

Meal 4	Portion Sizes	Fat	Calories	Carbs	Protein
TOTALS					

Satisfied after eating?	

Meal 5	Portion Sizes	Fat	Calories	Carbs	Protein
TOTALS					

Satisfied after eating?	

DAY #: _____

Meal 1	Portion Sizes	Fat	Calories	Carbs	Protein
TOTALS					
Satisfied after eating?					

Meal 2	Portion Sizes	Fat	Calories	Carbs	Protein
TOTALS					
Satisfied after eating?					

Notes

Meal 3	Portion Sizes	Fat	Calories	Carbs	Protein
TOTALS					

Satisfied after eating?

Meal 4	Portion Sizes	Fat	Calories	Carbs	Protein
TOTALS					

Satisfied after eating?

Meal 5	Portion Sizes	Fat	Calories	Carbs	Protein
TOTALS					

Satisfied after eating?

DAY #: _____

Meal 1	Portion Sizes	Fat	Calories	Carbs	Protein
TOTALS					
Satisfied after eating?					

Meal 2	Portion Sizes	Fat	Calories	Carbs	Protein
TOTALS					
Satisfied after eating?					

Notes

Meal 3	Portion Sizes	Fat	Calories	Carbs	Protein
TOTALS					

Satisfied after eating?		

Meal 4	Portion Sizes	Fat	Calories	Carbs	Protein
TOTALS					

Satisfied after eating?		

Meal 5	Portion Sizes	Fat	Calories	Carbs	Protein
TOTALS					

Satisfied after eating?		

DAY #:_____

Meal 1	Portion Sizes	Fat	Calories	Carbs	Protein
TOTALS					
Satisfied after eating?					

Meal 2	Portion Sizes	Fat	Calories	Carbs	Protein
TOTALS					
Satisfied after eating?					

Notes

Meal 3	Portion Sizes	Fat	Calories	Carbs	Protein
TOTALS					

Satisfied after eating?	

Meal 4	Portion Sizes	Fat	Calories	Carbs	Protein
TOTALS					

Satisfied after eating?	

Meal 5	Portion Sizes	Fat	Calories	Carbs	Protein
TOTALS					

Satisfied after eating?	

DAY #: _____

Meal 1	Portion Sizes	Fat	Calories	Carbs	Protein
TOTALS					

Satisfied after eating? (..................)

Meal 2	Portion Sizes	Fat	Calories	Carbs	Protein
TOTALS					

Satisfied after eating? (..................)

Notes

Meal 3	Portion Sizes	Fat	Calories	Carbs	Protein
TOTALS					

Satisfied after eating?

Meal 4	Portion Sizes	Fat	Calories	Carbs	Protein
TOTALS					

Satisfied after eating?

Meal 5	Portion Sizes	Fat	Calories	Carbs	Protein
TOTALS					

Satisfied after eating?

DAY #: _____

Meal 1	Portion Sizes	Fat	Calories	Carbs	Protein
TOTALS					
Satisfied after eating?					

Meal 2	Portion Sizes	Fat	Calories	Carbs	Protein
TOTALS					
Satisfied after eating?					

Notes

Meal 3	Portion Sizes	Fat	Calories	Carbs	Protein
TOTALS					
Satisfied after eating?					

Meal 4	Portion Sizes	Fat	Calories	Carbs	Protein
TOTALS					
Satisfied after eating?					

Meal 5	Portion Sizes	Fat	Calories	Carbs	Protein
TOTALS					
Satisfied after eating?					

DAY #:_____

Meal 1	Portion Sizes	Fat	Calories	Carbs	Protein
TOTALS					
Satisfied after eating?					

Meal 2	Portion Sizes	Fat	Calories	Carbs	Protein
TOTALS					
Satisfied after eating?					

Notes

Meal 3	Portion Sizes	Fat	Calories	Carbs	Protein
TOTALS					

Satisfied after eating?

Meal 4	Portion Sizes	Fat	Calories	Carbs	Protein
TOTALS					

Satisfied after eating?

Meal 5	Portion Sizes	Fat	Calories	Carbs	Protein
TOTALS					

Satisfied after eating?

DAY #:_____

Meal 1	Portion Sizes	Fat	Calories	Carbs	Protein
TOTALS					
Satisfied after eating?					

Meal 2	Portion Sizes	Fat	Calories	Carbs	Protein
TOTALS					
Satisfied after eating?					

Notes

Meal 3	Portion Sizes	Fat	Calories	Carbs	Protein
TOTALS					
Satisfied after eating?					

Meal 4	Portion Sizes	Fat	Calories	Carbs	Protein
TOTALS					
Satisfied after eating?					

Meal 5	Portion Sizes	Fat	Calories	Carbs	Protein
TOTALS					
Satisfied after eating?					

DAY #: _____

Meal 1	Portion Sizes	Fat	Calories	Carbs	Protein
TOTALS					
Satisfied after eating?					

Meal 2	Portion Sizes	Fat	Calories	Carbs	Protein
TOTALS					
Satisfied after eating?					

Notes

Meal 3	Portion Sizes		Fat	Calories	Carbs	Protein
TOTALS						
Satisfied after eating?						

Meal 4	Portion Sizes		Fat	Calories	Carbs	Protein
TOTALS						
Satisfied after eating?						

Meal 5	Portion Sizes		Fat	Calories	Carbs	Protein
TOTALS						
Satisfied after eating?